LOW CHOLESTEROL DIET

COOKBOOK

FOR

VEGETARIANS

*Delicious recipes to achieve
low fat and healthy living*

Susan Snow

Copyright © 2024 [Susan Snow)]

TABLE OF CONTENTS

Hydration : Staying adequately doused is essential. Water is a calorie-free option that aids digestion and supports overall health. Meal Planning Plan reflections in advance to ensure a balanced input of nutrients. Including a variety of foods helps with nutritional deficiencies. Supplementation Depending on individual conditions, consider supplementing with vitamins like B12, vitamin D, and omega- 3 adipose acids. Consult a Dietitian personalized advice from a registered dietitian ensures that nutrient conditions are met while following a low- fat invertebrate diet. Flash back, the key to a successful low- fat invertebrate diet is balance. By combining a variety of plant- predicated foods and being of fat sources, individualities can achieve

INTRODUCTION

Once upon a time in the bustling city of Greenleaf, a group of health-conscious friends decided to embark on a journey to embrace a low-cholesterol diet for vegetarians. The lively bunch, led by a nutrition-savvy enthusiast named Lily, gathered in her cozy kitchen to explore the vibrant world of plant-based goodness.

Their adventure began with colorful trips to the local farmers' market, where they marveled at the array of fresh fruits, vegetables, and whole grains. As they filled their baskets with kale, quinoa, and a rainbow of produce, they felt a sense of excitement about the delicious possibilities ahead.

In Lily's kitchen, the group experimented with innovative recipes that replaced traditional high-cholesterol ingredients with wholesome alternatives. Tofu stir-fries, chickpea burgers, and avocado salads became their staples, each bite bursting with flavor and nutritional benefits.

As the friends swapped stories of their dietary discoveries, they noticed improvements in their well-being. Energy levels soared, and the once-dreaded cholesterol numbers began to drop. Encouraged by their success, they even hosted a vegetarian potluck, inviting the entire neighborhood to savor the delights of their low-cholesterol creations.

Word spread quickly, and soon the city of Greenleaf became a hub for health-conscious living. The local restaurants embraced the trend, introducing delicious low-cholesterol options to cater to the growing demand. The community flourished as residents embraced the benefits of a plant-based lifestyle, fostering a sense of well-being and connection.

And so, in the heart of Greenleaf, a story of health, friendship, and culinary exploration unfolded—one low-cholesterol meal at a time. The city's journey towards a healthier lifestyle served as inspiration for other communities, proving that a vegetarian diet rich in nutrients could lead to a fulfilling and vibrant life.

CHAPTER ONE

Vegetarians

Individuals who follow a diet that primarily excludes meat and, in some cases, other animal products. This dietary choice can be motivated by various factors, including ethical, environmental, and health considerations.

1. Types of Vegetarians:

Lacto-ovo vegetarians: Eat eggs and dairy products, but stay away from fish, poultry, and meat.

Eat dairy products, but stay away from fish, poultry, pork, and eggs if you're a *lacto-vegetarian.*

Eggs are permissible for *ovo-vegetarians,* while dairy, fish, poultry, and meat are not.

Vegans: Steer clear of anything that comes from animals, including dairy, eggs, and sometimes honey.

2. Ethical and Environmental Considerations:

Vegetarianism is largely motivated by ethical concerns about animal welfare. They may object to industrial farming practices and the way animals are handled in the meat business.
Since the production of meat is frequently associated with deforestation, water use, and greenhouse gas emissions, environmental **sustainability** is another driving force.

3. Health Considerations:

A well-balanced vegetarian diet can provide essential nutrients like vitamins, minerals, fiber, and antioxidants.
Studies suggest that vegetarians may have lower risks of certain health issues, such as heart disease, high blood pressure, and type 2 diabetes.
However, it's crucial for vegetarians to pay attention to specific nutrients like B12, iron, calcium, and omega-3 fatty acids, which are commonly found in animal products.

4. Challenges and Misconceptions:

One challenge vegetarians face is ensuring they obtain enough protein, as many protein-rich sources are animal-based. However, plant-based protein options are abundant and diverse.
Some people may hold misconceptions about vegetarian diets, such as assuming they lack protein or are inherently deficient. With proper planning, vegetarians can meet their nutritional needs.
5. Vegetarianism Worldwide:

The prevalence of vegetarianism varies globally, influenced by cultural, religious, and socioeconomic factors.
In some countries, vegetarianism is deeply rooted in cultural or religious practices, while in others, it's a personal choice driven by health or environmental concerns.

6. Growing Popularity and Trends:

Over the years, there has been a noticeable increase in the popularity of vegetarianism and veganism. This rise is attributed to a growing awareness of ethical and environmental issues, as well as health consciousness.Restaurants and food industries are adapting to this trend by offering more vegetarian and plant-based options.

7. Vegetarianism and Balanced Nutrition:

Planning a well-balanced vegetarian diet involves incorporating a variety of fruits, vegetables, whole grains, legumes, nuts, and seeds.
Education on nutrition is essential for vegetarians to make informed choices and avoid potential nutritional deficiencies.
In conclusion, vegetarianism is a diverse and evolving lifestyle choice influenced by ethical, environmental, and health considerations. As awareness continues to grow, so does the availability of resources and support for those choosing a plant-based diet.

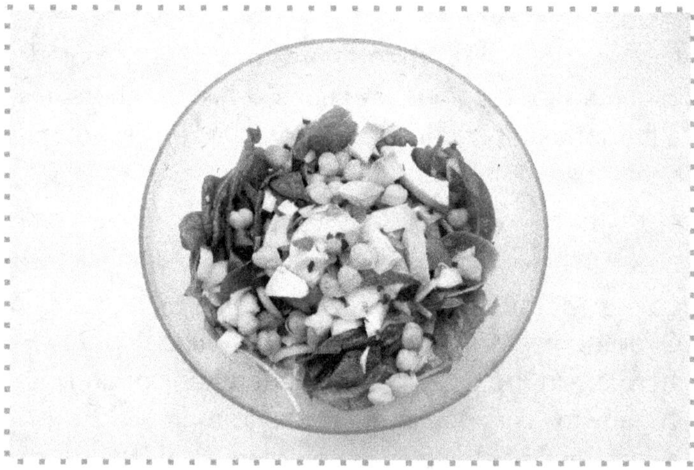

CHAPTER TWO

Cholesterol and it's role

Cholesterol plays a crucial role in the body, serving as a structural component of cell membranes and a precursor for essential hormones. While dietary cholesterol is often associated with animal products, *it's important to note that vegetarians can also be affected by cholesterol levels, albeit in a different way.*

Vegetarian diets typically exclude or limit animal products, which are primary sources of dietary cholesterol. As a result, many vegetarians often have lower levels of LDL (low-density lipoprotein) or "bad" cholesterol compared to non-vegetarians. This can be attributed to the absence of saturated fats and cholesterol-rich foods found in meat and dairy products.

However, it's crucial for vegetarians to pay attention to other dietary factors that can influence cholesterol levels. While plant-based diets can be rich in fiber, antioxidants, and unsaturated fats, certain vegetarian foods may contribute to elevated cholesterol if consumed excessively. For example, highly processed plant-based products, fried foods, and those high in refined sugars can impact cholesterol levels negatively.

To maintain a healthy cholesterol profile, vegetarians are encouraged to focus on whole, minimally processed foods such as *fruits, vegetables, whole grains, legumes, nuts, and seeds.* These foods are not only cholesterol-free but also provide essential nutrients that support overall cardiovascular health.

Moreover, incorporating omega-3 fatty acids from plant sources like flaxseeds, chia seeds, and walnuts can contribute to a favorable lipid profile. These healthy fats have been associated with lower triglyceride levels and may help raise HDL (high-density lipoprotein) or "good" cholesterol.

CHAPTER THREE

The goal of good living is to consume less cholesterol, which is essential for heart health. Limiting saturated and trans fats—found in processed meals and animal products—is one way to do this. Place a focus on lean proteins, whole grains, fruits, and vegetables. Fish and other seafood are good providers of omega-3 fatty acids. Consider portion proportions and use techniques such as steaming or baking. Frequent exercise enhances a low-cholesterol way of life. For tailored advice, always speak with a healthcare professional.

A vegetarian diet emphasizes plant-based meals and excludes meat, poultry, and fish. Vegetarians need to include a range of fruits, vegetables, grains, legumes, nuts, and seeds in their meals to guarantee proper nutrition.

Low- fat diets for insectivores concentrate on reducing overall fat input while emphasizing plant- predicated foods. Incorporating a variety of nutrient- thick fruits, vegetables, whole grains, legumes, and spare plant- predicated proteins is pivotal. analogous diets aim to promote heart health, weight operation, and overall well- being.

plant- predicated Protein Sources conclude for legumes like lentils, chickpeas, and tire. Tofu and tempeh are excellent protein-rich options with lower fat content. Include quinoa, brown rice, and whole grains for sustained energy.

Healthy Fats While reducing overall fat input, it's vital to include sources of healthy fats like avocados, nuts, and seeds in temperance. Use olive oil painting oil or canola oil painting oil for cooking in controlled amounts.

Dairy Alternatives Choose low- fat or fat-free dairy druthers like almond milk, soy milk, or oat milk. Greek yogurt or low- fat yogurt can be part of the diet for added protein.

Emphasize Fruits and Vegetables Aim for a colorful array of fruits and vegetables to ensure a broad spectrum of nutrients. These foods are naturally low in fat and high in essential vitamins and minerals.

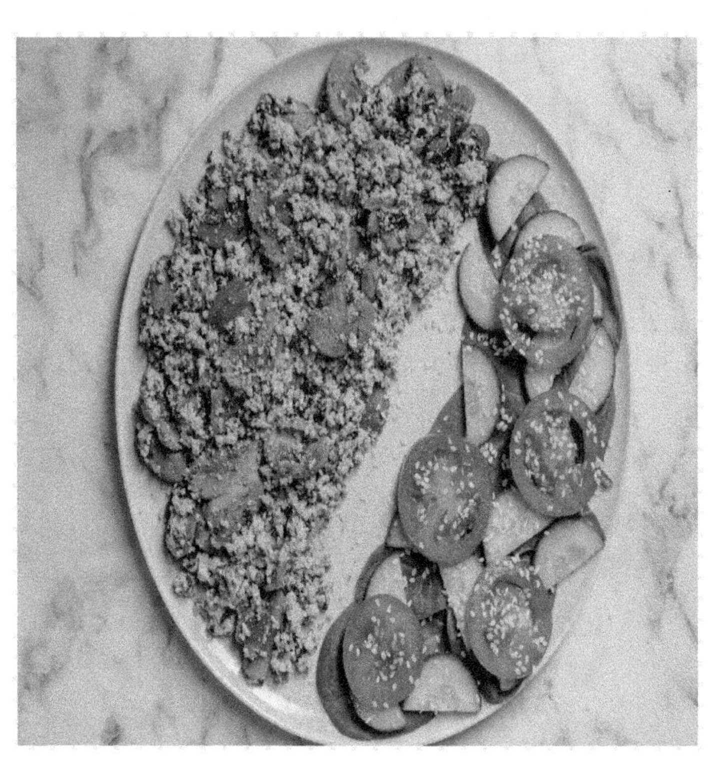

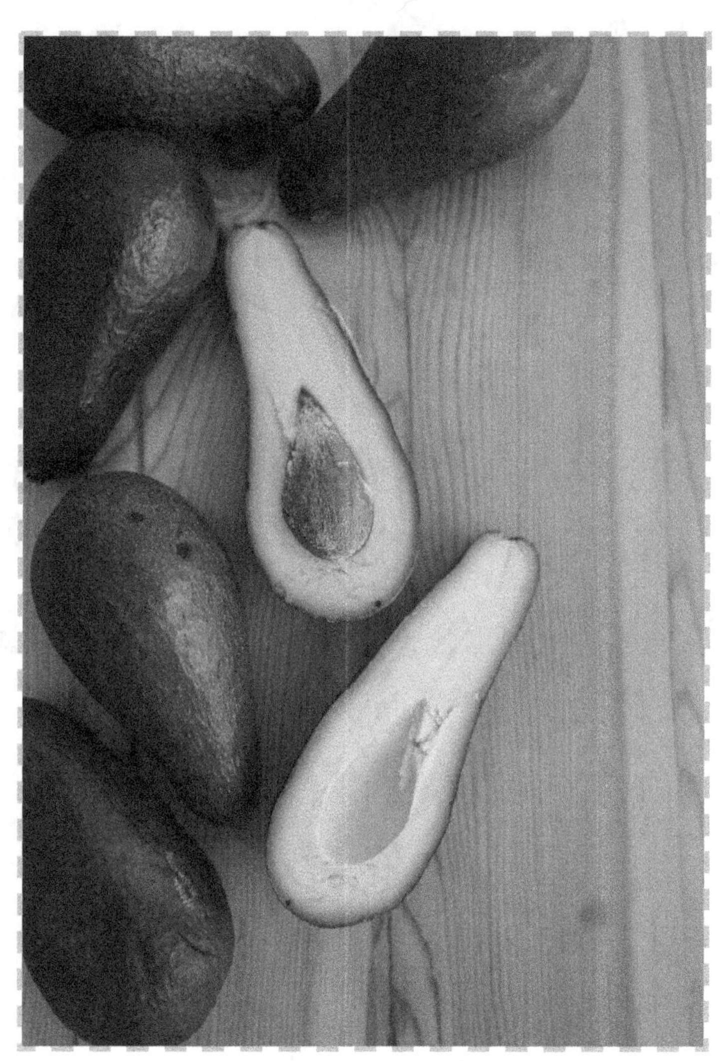

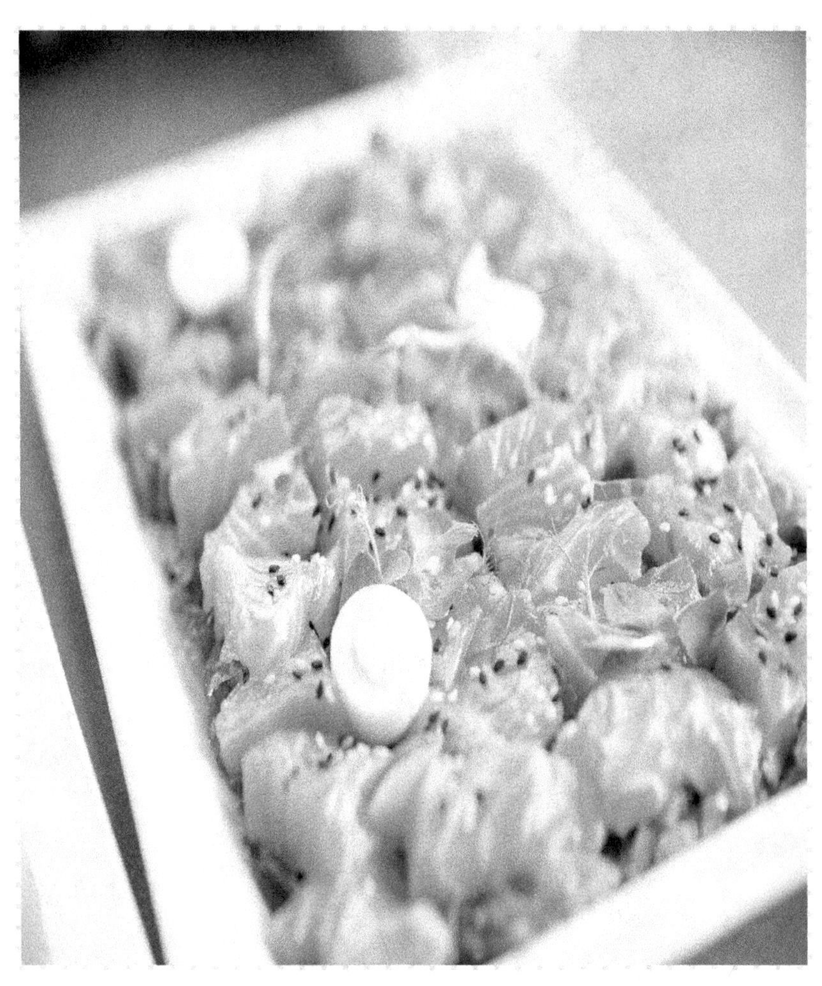

CHAPTER FOUR

Crucial components

Protein Sources:

Legumes that are high in protein include chickpeas, lentils, and beans.
The two versatile plant-based protein options are tofu and tempeh.
Both quinoa and soy products offer full proteins.

Foods High in Iron:

Dark greens like spinach and kale are good sources of iron.
Legumes, fortified cereals, and chickpeas are additional sources of iron.

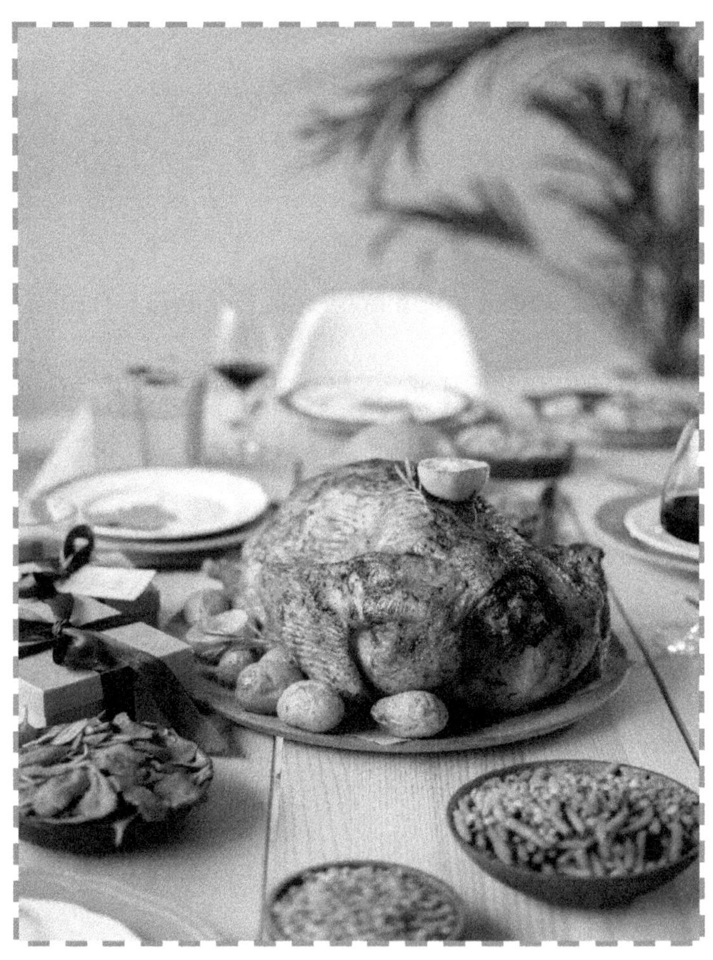

Foods rich in Iron

Calcium Intake:

Plant-based milk alternatives such fortified soy,
almond, or oat milk satisfy calcium requirements.
Other foods high in calcium include leafy greens,
tofu, and fortified orange juice.

Vitamin B12:

Fortified foods including cereals, plant-based milk,
and nutritional yeast are good sources of vitamin
B12.
Since the primary source of this vitamin is animal
food, consider taking supplements if needed.

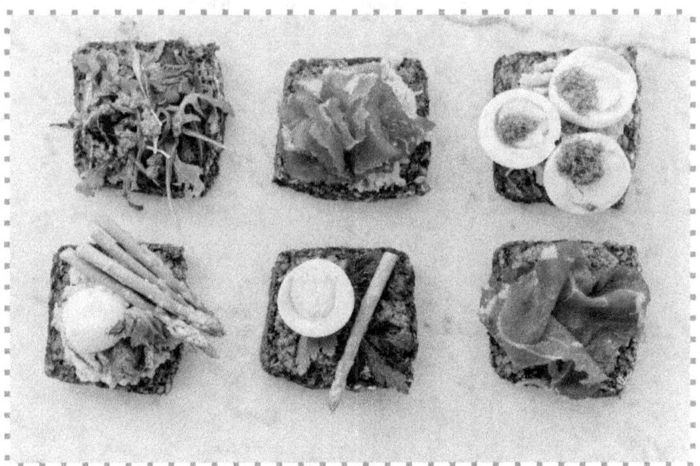

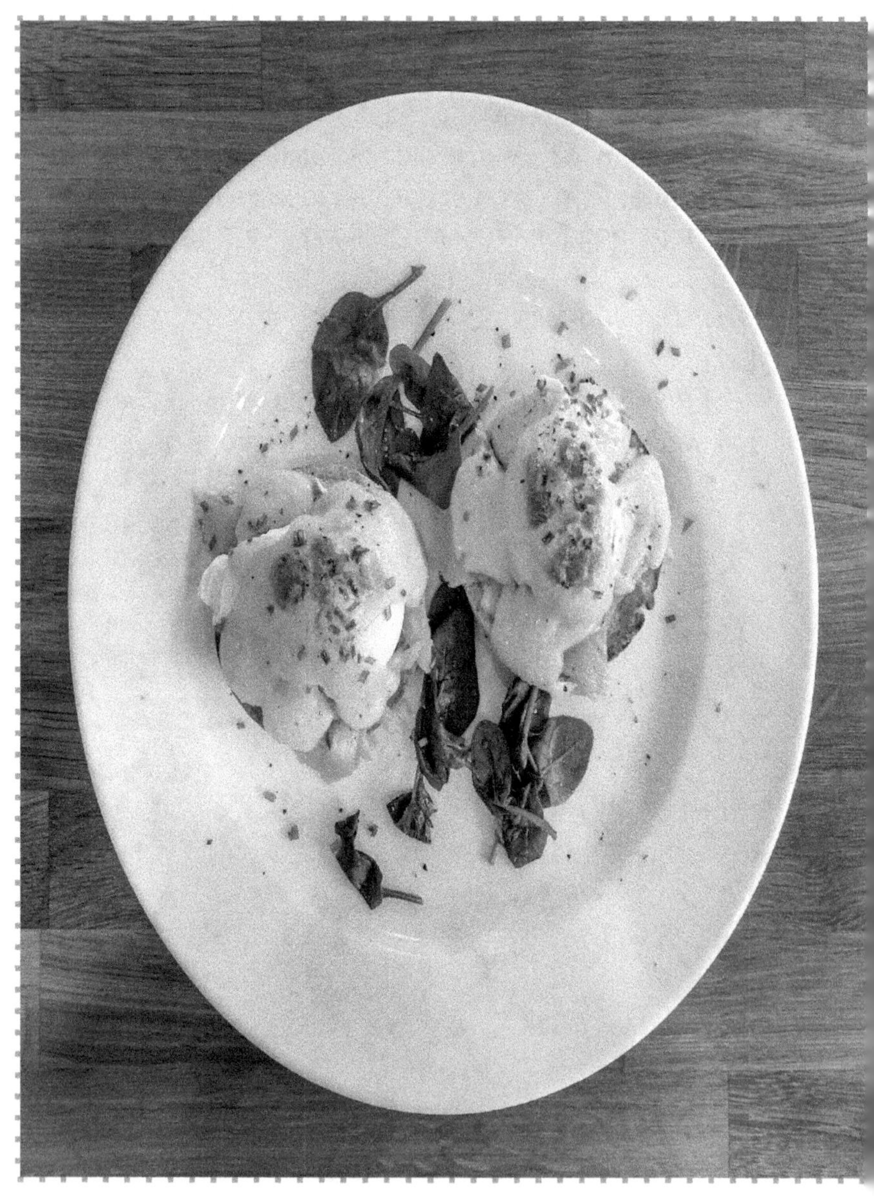

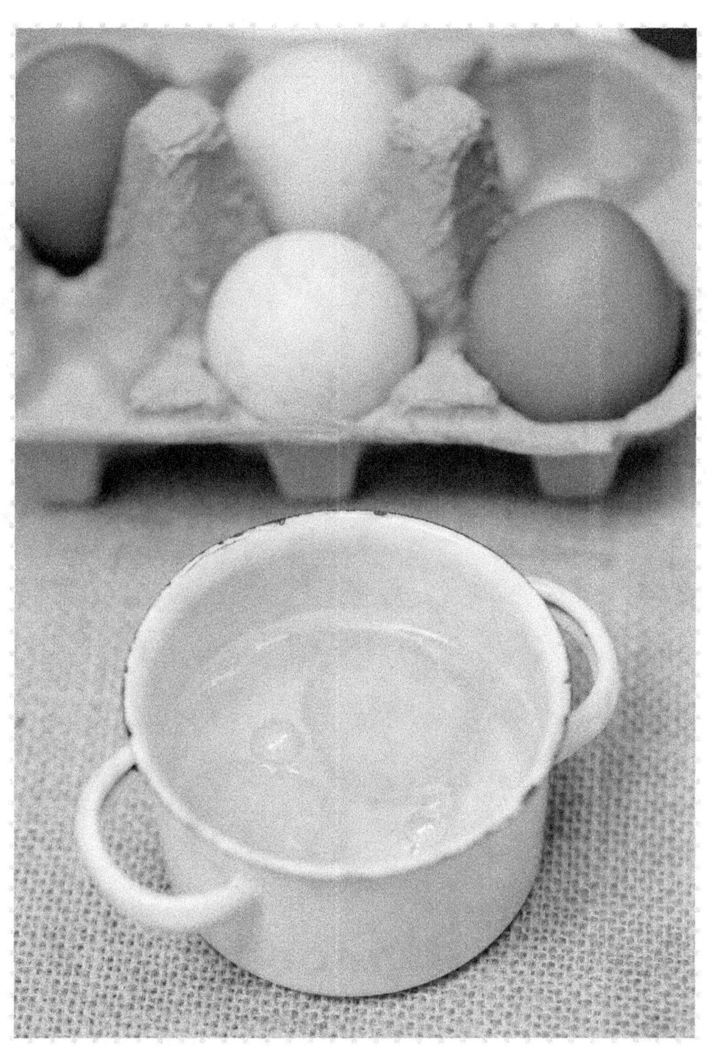

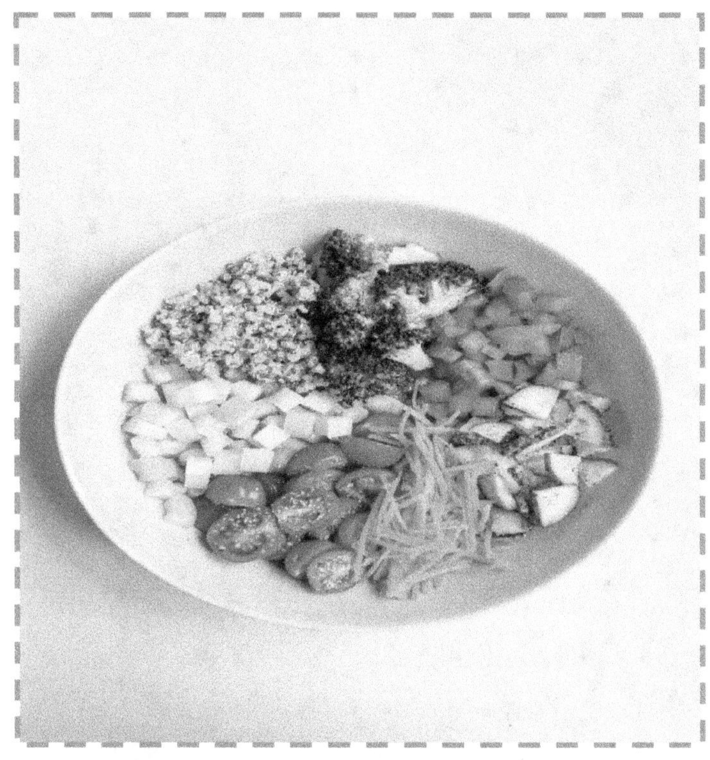

Calcium rich foods

CHAPTER FIVE

Control of Portion:

A healthy weight should be maintained by watching portion sizes because being overweight might raise cholesterol.

Portion Sizes Being apprehensive of portion sizes helps manage sweet input and contributes to weight control. lower, frequent refections can help maintain energy situations throughout the day. Limit Reused Foods Reused amenable products may contain sheltered fats and complements. Whole, minimally reused foods are preferable for a nutrient-rich diet.

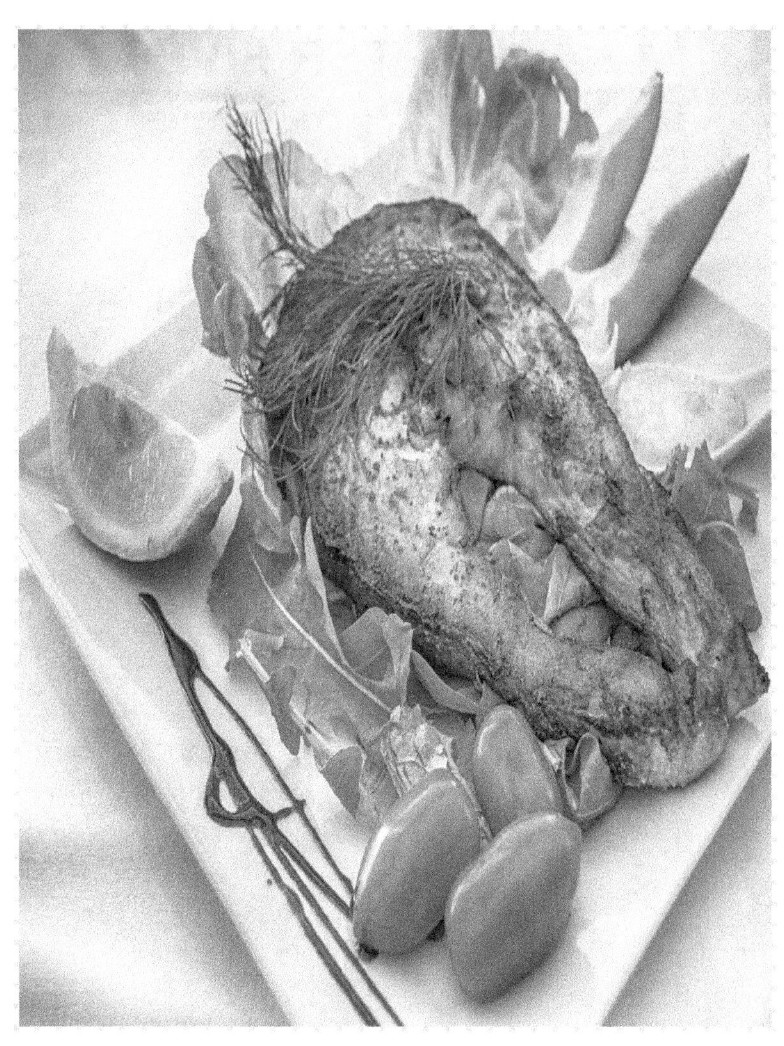

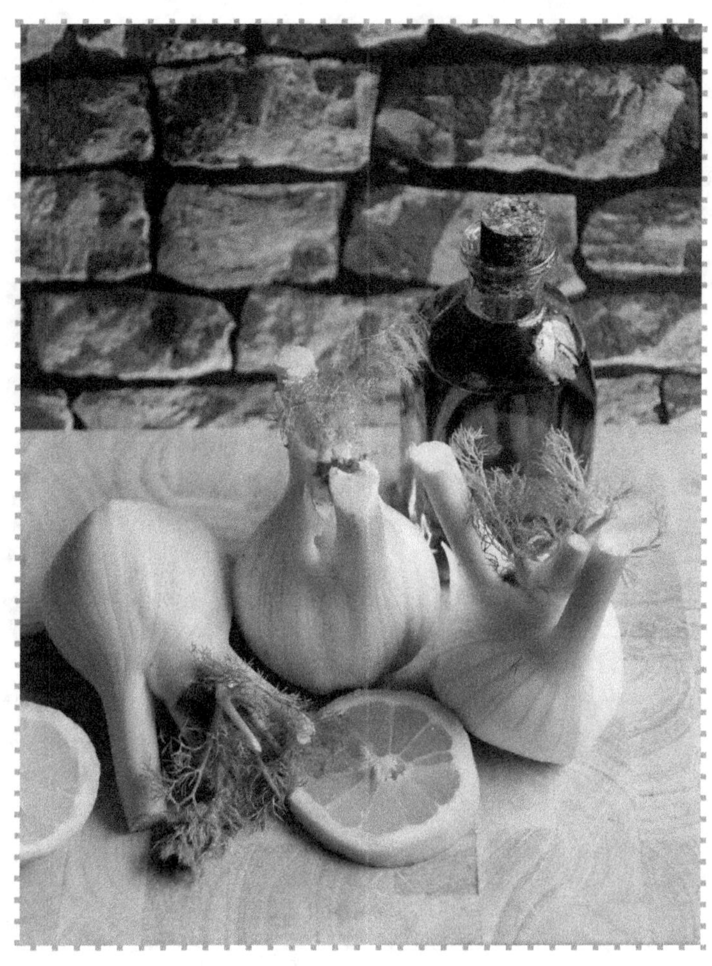

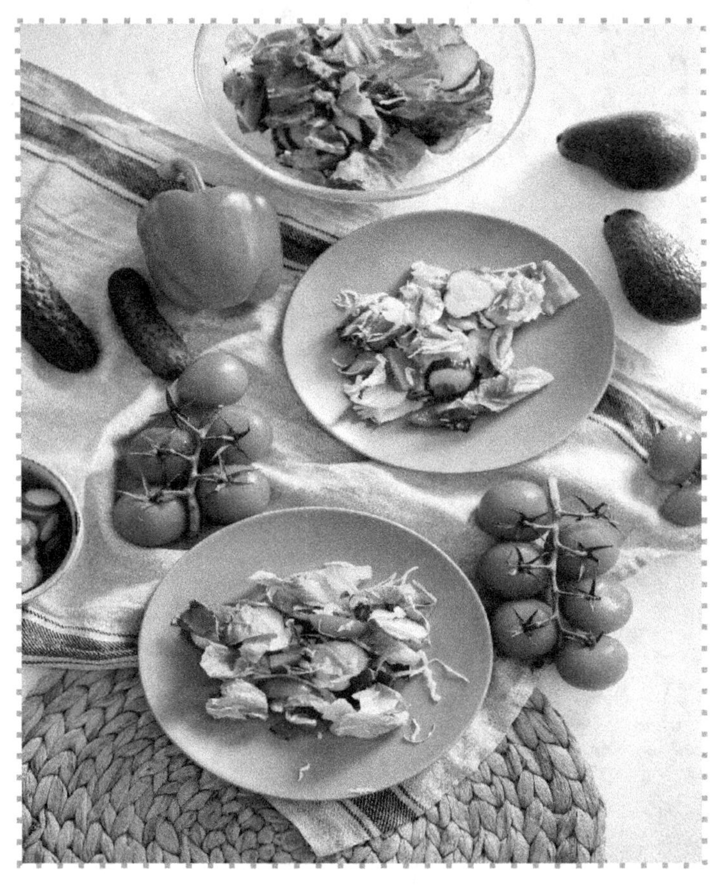

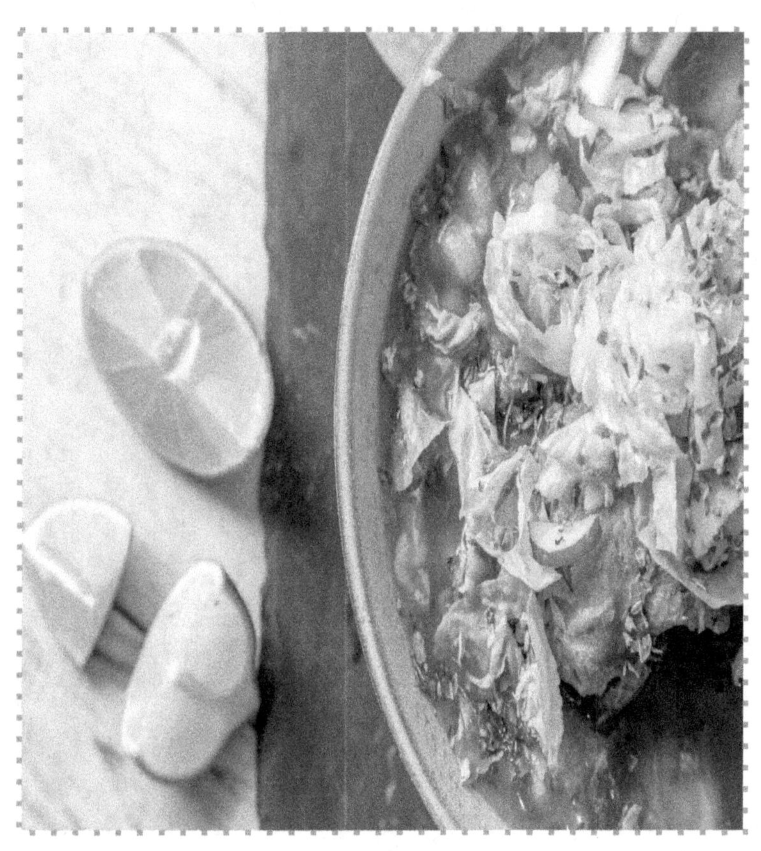

Hydration : Staying adequately doused
is essential. Water is a calorie-free
option that aids digestion and supports
overall health. **Meal Planning Plan
reflections** in advance to ensure a
balanced input of nutrients. Including a
variety of foods helps with nutritional
deficiencies. Supplementation
Depending on individual conditions,
consider supplementing with vitamins
like B12, vitamin D, and omega- 3
adipose acids. **Consult a Dietitian**
personalized advice from a registered
dietitian ensures that nutrient conditions
are met while following a low- fat
invertebrate diet. Flash back, the key to
a successful low- fat invertebrate diet is
balance. By combining a variety of
plant- predicated foods and being of fat
sources, individualities can achieve their
nutritional pretensions while enjoying a
luscious and satisfying diet.

CHAPTER SIX

Daily diets suggestions for healthy living

FOR BREAKFAST: Oatmeal with a few almonds and berries on top

Toast made with whole grains,avocado and tomatoes

FOR LUNCH: mixed veggies and quinoa salad topped with a vinaigrette dressing.

Whole grain bread served alongside lentil soup.

FOR DINNER: Roasted vegetables paired with grilled tempeh or tofu.

Curry with chicken peas and brown rice

Certainly! Here are a few delicious recipes tailored for a low-fat vegetarian diet:

Toss quinoa with roasted vegetables like bell peppers, cherry tomatoes, and zucchini.

Dress with a light vinaigrette made from lemon juice, olive oil, and herbs.

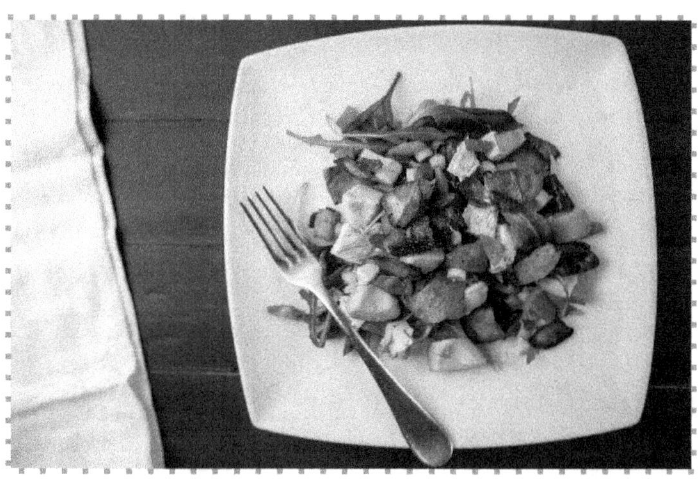

Stuffed Bell Peppers:

Mix cooked brown rice with black beans, corn, diced tomatoes, and spices.

Stuff the mixture into halved bell peppers.

Bake until peppers are tender.

Spaghetti Squash Primavera:

Roast spaghetti squash until tender, then scrape out the strands.

Sauté colorful vegetables like broccoli, cherry tomatoes, and bell peppers.

Toss with the spaghetti squash and a light marinara sauce.

Lentil and Vegetable Soup:

Cook lentils with a variety of vegetables like carrots, celery, and spinach.

Season with garlic, cumin, and coriander for added flavor.

Cauliflower and Chickpea Curry:

Sauté cauliflower and chickpeas with onions, garlic, and ginger.

Simmer in a light coconut milk-based curry sauce with turmeric and cumin.

Zucchini Noodles with Pesto:

Spiralize zucchini into noodles and sauté lightly.

Toss with homemade basil pesto made with pine nuts, garlic, and a touch of olive oil.

Sweet Potato and Black Bean Burgers:

Mash cooked sweet potatoes and mix with black beans, breadcrumbs, and spices.

Form into patties and bake until golden brown.

Mushroom and Spinach Omelette:

Whisk together eggs and pour into a pan.

Fill with sautéed mushrooms, spinach, and a sprinkle of low-fat cheese.

Cucumber Avocado Sushi Rolls:

Use cucumber strips instead of rice to roll with avocado, carrots, and bell peppers.

Serve with low-sodium soy sauce.

Chickpea Salad Wrap:

Mash chickpeas and mix with diced cucumbers, tomatoes, and red onion.

Spread the mixture onto a whole-grain wrap and roll it up.

Remember to focus on whole, unprocessed foods, and use herbs and spices for flavor without relying on excessive fats. Adjust portion sizes according to individual dietary needs.

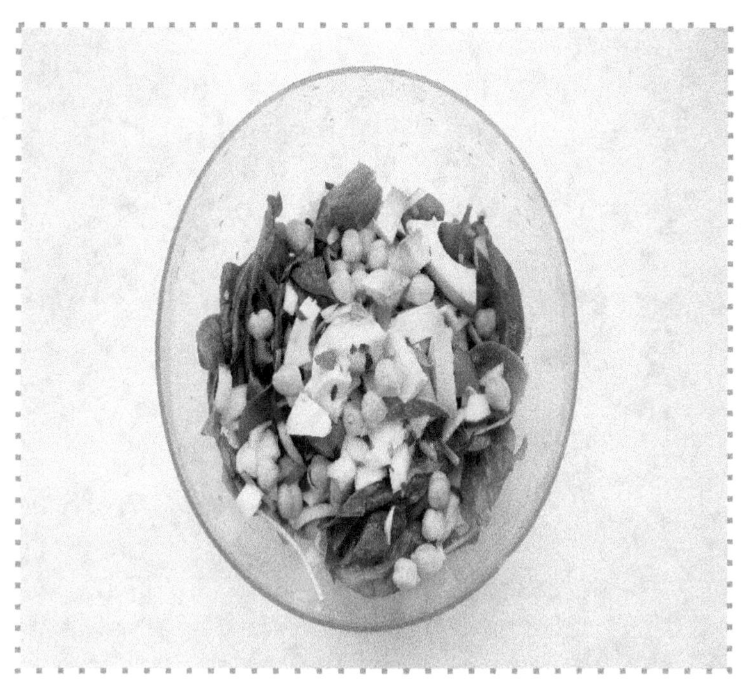

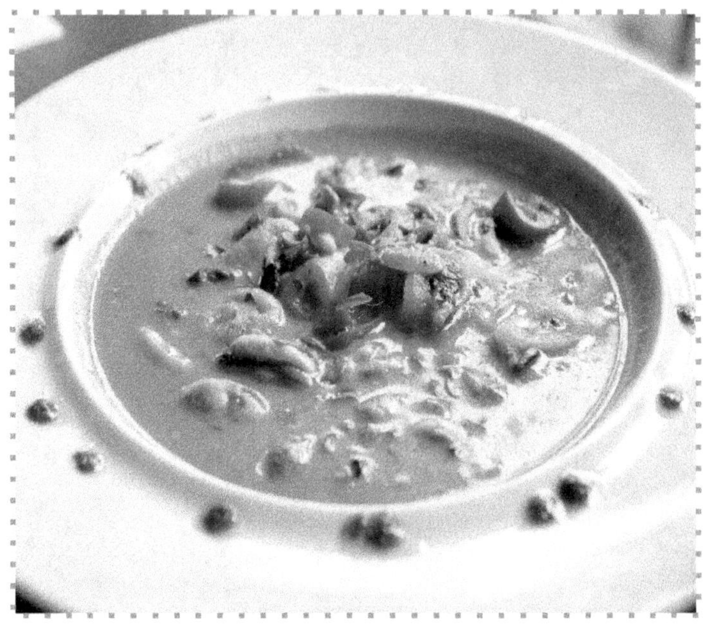

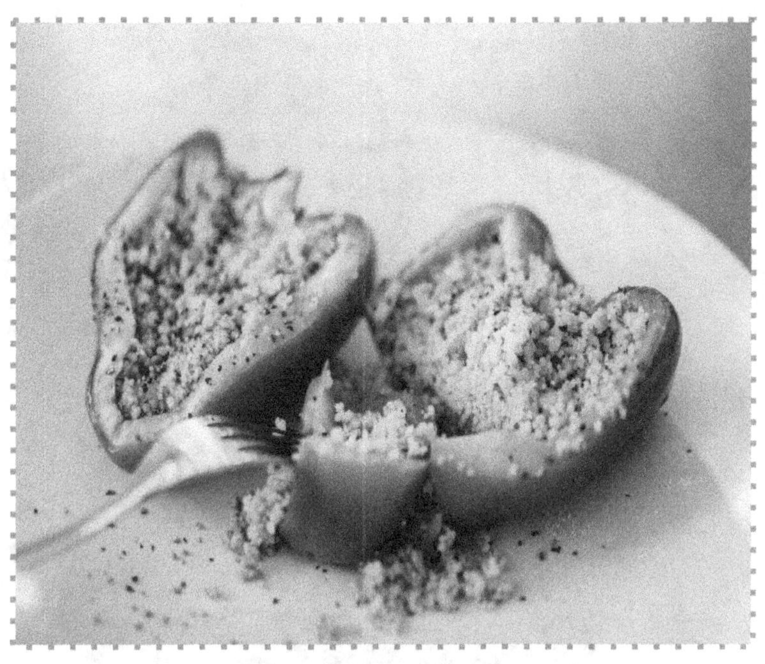

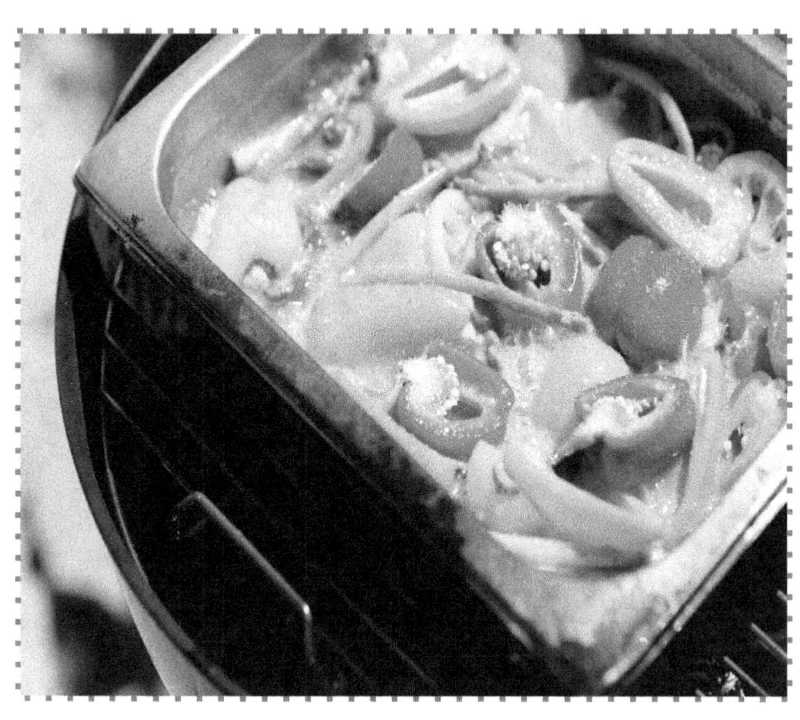

CHAPTER SEVEN

Lifestyle Suggestions

Variety Is Essential:

A wide variety of vibrant fruits and vegetables guarantees a wide range of nutrients.
Change up your diet to include all the necessary vitamins and minerals.

Organizing Meals:

Meal plans should incorporate a range of veggies, healthy fats, carbohydrates, and proteins.
Try out several recipes to maintain an intriguing and well-balanced diet.
Drinking plenty of water

Make sure you're getting enough water to help with digestion and general wellness.

Having a Nutritionist Consultation:

Consult a dietitian for advice on customizing a vegetarian diet to meet your needs.
Check-ups on a regular basis can guarantee that nutritional needs are being satisfied.
Recall that a well-planned vegetarian diet can supply all the nutrients required for a healthy way of living. It's critical to be knowledgeable, consider dietary needs, and make any dietary adjustme

Consistent Exercise:

Engaging in physical activity can enhance heart health overall and increase HDL (good) cholesterol.

Track Your Cholesterol Amounts:

Get your cholesterol checked on a regular basis by medical professionals to monitor your progress and make any necessary corrections.
A vegetarian diet that is well-planned, full of foods high in nutrients and low in fats, can help to keep cholesterol levels within normal ranges and improve cardiovascular health in general.

CONCLUSION

A low-cholesterol diet for vegetarians can have several positive health implications. By emphasizing plant-based foods, individuals can reduce their intake of saturated fats and cholesterol, contributing to better heart health. The conclusion drawn from adopting such a diet often involves improvements in lipid profiles, including lower levels of LDL (low-density lipoprotein) cholesterol, commonly known as the "bad" cholesterol.

Vegetarian diets rich in fruits, vegetables, whole grains, legumes, and nuts offer a myriad of benefits. These foods are not only naturally low in cholesterol but also high in fiber, antioxidants, and various essential nutrients. The cumulative effect of these dietary elements is a decreased risk of cardiovascular diseases. Studies have suggested that adopting a vegetarian lifestyle may be associated with lower blood pressure, reduced inflammation, and improved overall cardiovascular health.

Moreover, low-cholesterol vegetarian diets may contribute to weight management, another crucial factor in heart health. Many plant-based foods are lower in calories and unhealthy fats, making it easier for individuals to maintain a healthy weight. Weight management, in turn, plays a pivotal role in preventing obesity-related complications, including high cholesterol levels.

It's important to note that while a vegetarian diet can be beneficial for heart health, the quality of food choices matters. A well-balanced and nutrient-dense vegetarian diet is key to reaping the full spectrum of health benefits. This includes incorporating a variety of plant-based protein sources, such as beans, lentils, tofu, and nuts, to ensure adequate protein intake.

In conclusion, adopting a low-cholesterol vegetarian diet holds promise for enhancing cardiovascular health. It not only addresses concerns related to cholesterol levels but also promotes overall well-being through the consumption of nutrient-rich, plant-based foods. However, as with any dietary approach, it's crucial for individuals to make informed and balanced choices to ensure they meet their nutritional needs. Consulting with a healthcare professional or a registered dietitian can provide personalized guidance for those considering or already following a low-cholesterol vegetarian diet.